Simply Handmade

Beauty & Skincare Handcrafted Recipes

Kimberly Hodge

Contents

Introduction

Today we have a tendency to treat our self care as an afterthought. We grab a bottle of lotion or shampoo and conditioner at the local grocery or pharmacy without another thought, not bothering to read the ingredients. Who has time, am I right?

Most spend more time focusing their attention on what we put into our bodies, but now what we are putting on it.

It wasn't until my eyelids swelled shut that I realized I was having an allergic reaction to the shampoo and conditioner that I was using that I purchased from a well known bath and body retail store. I decided to research the ingredients and I was shocked! The harmful ingredients were full of chemicals and dyes. No wonder I had an allergic reaction! I needed to make a change now.

I started researching how to make my own handmade all-natural products, and I was hooked! Many of the ingredients I already had in my own kitchen. I was able to whip up a variety of wholesome products for myself, friends, and family.

Disclaimer

The authors and publisher are not responsible for any misuse of the information in this book, nor are they responsible for any allergic or adverse reactions. The safe and proper use of the recipes, ingredients, and equipment, is the sole responsibility of the individual using them.

The advise and suggestions in this book should not, in any way, be interpreted as medical advice, and any health concerns the user may have, should be addressed by a qualified medical practitioner.

The author and publisher have made every effort to ensure the accuracy of the information in this book, and assume no responsibility for errors, omissions, inaccuracies, or inconsistencies.

Book Structure

In this book I have made every effort to make clear, concise, easy to follow, instructions so that the reader can practice and learn at their own pace. The structure of the book is made up of five chapters:

Chapter 1: Basic Skincare - In this section we will cover the benefits of making your own beauty and skincare products, the anatomy of the skin, skin types, and basic skincare routines.

Chapter 2: Getting Started - The materials and equipment needed, and the techniques you need to learn. Rushing straight into making recipes is tempting, however, take the time to read and learn the skills you will need in order to avoid making costly mistakes. This step offers the all-important advice on not only how to make the products safely, but how to store them to ensure they have the best possible shelf life.

Chapter 3: Home Apothecary - Reviews the common ingredients used in recipes such as; Butters, Essential Oils, Herbs & Flowers, Oils, Wax, and other supplies.

Chapter 4: Skincare Recipes - This section is subdivided into recipes for your face, body, hair, and baby, so you can begin to whip up your own luscious products.

Chapter 5: Bonus Recipes - In this section you will find recipes for use in your home.

Chapter 6: Resources - This section provides valuable

resource information on the necessary supplies that you will need in order to begin your journey.

Chapter 1: Why Make Your Own Products?

<u>First off, you know exactly what's in them!</u> Have you ever looked at the ingredients listed on one of your beauty products? Look at the ingredients listed on your shampoo bottle, lotion bottle, or your make-up products. Go ahead – I'll wait.

See what I mean? I can't even pronounce some of the chemical ingredients listed!

<u>Let's look at just a few chemicals listed on some of these products:</u>

Fragrance:

Fragrances are complex combinations of natural and/or man-made substances that are added to many consumer products to give them a pleasurable smell.

If a cosmetic is marketed to retail consumers, it must have a list of ingredients. In most cases, each ingredient must be listed individually. But under U.S. regulations, fragrance ingredients can be listed collectively simply as "Fragrance."

Fragrance and flavor formulas can be a complex mixture of many different natural and/or man-made chemical ingredients. These "formulas" are the kinds of cosmetic components that can be considered "trade secrets", therefore, a company may list all the ingredients (sometimes in the hundreds) as a fragrance and claim them to be a "trade secret".

This is not good for the end consumer! Especially for those of us that are very sensitive or have allergies. By allowing the manufacturers to list ingredients as "fragrance", they are bypassing the regulation to list all ingredients allowing us to make safe and informed decisions.

Below you will find just a **<u>few</u>** examples in some of our bath body, beauty, and cleaning products:

Hand Cream:

Butylphenyl Methylpropional – (p-tert-butyl-alpha-methylhydrocinnamic aldehyde) is colorless to pale yellow liquid with a powerful, floral-fresh odor.

Dimethicone – (polydimethylsiloxane) is a silicon-based polymer that is a man-made synthetic molecule.

Mascara:

Ammonium Acrylates Copolymer – (Acrylates Copolymer) is a general term for copolymers of two or more monomers consisting of acrylic acid, methacrylic acid or one of their simple esters.

Propylene glycol – (1,2-propanediol) is a man-made synthetic organic alcohol. Propylene glycol is one of the most widely used ingredients in cosmetics and personal care products, where it also serves as a viscosity degreasing agent, solvent, and a fragrance ingredient.

Bubble Bath:

Sodium Laureth Sulfate - ingredients function as surfactants and are used as cleansing agents. Can be found in shampoos, household cleaning products, and even garage floor cleaners.

Spray Fragrance and Perfumes:

Petrolatum – (white petrolatum) belongs to a class of chemicals referred to as hydrocarbons, a group of compounds containing only carbon and hydrogen.

Hydrocarbons are generally derived from petroleum. A great majority of consumer products used worldwide, including plastic bottles to automobile tires.

Butane – (Butane, Isobutane, Propane and Isopentane) They are volatile substances derived from petroleum and natural gas. These ingredients are found in cosmetics and personal care products as a replacement for chlorofluorocarbons, or CFC propellants, and some have been found to have negative effects on the environment.

These are just a few of the examples of ingredients listed in our personal care products, not to mention our cleaning products that we use each day.

When you make your own products, there's no question what ingredients are in it!

In addition to the above ingredients **look out for talc, phthalates and parabens.**

OK, back to why you should make your own products!

The second reason is that it's cheaper! Some brands of beauty products can cost you hundreds of dollars. You can make a better version at home for a fraction of the cost. Saving you hundreds, if not thousands of dollars a year! Put that savings aside and take a vacation, redecorate your home, re-invest in your business, or put it away for a rainy day!

<u>Third, let's get back to nature!</u> Does it make any sense to buy a product full of chemicals that promotes that it's added natural ingredients? Why not just use the natural product instead?

<u>Does this make any sense to you?</u>

Dish detergent now made with all-natural lemons

Lemonade Drink with artificial lemon flavor

<u>Nope. Didn't to me either!</u>

Exactly why are we drinking artificial lemon flavors and cleaning our dishes with all-natural lemons? What is going on with that?

Let's just put a stop to the insanity and make it pure and simple - **<u>and safer</u>**!

Benefits

There are many reasons to make your own beauty and skincare products.

Some of the most important reasons include:

- **All-Natural Ingredients**
- **Small Batches**
- **Vegan & Gluten Free**
- **Cruelty Free, No Animal Testing**
- **Customizable**
- **Creative Packaging**
- **Saves Money**
- **Non-Toxic, Chemical & Synthetic Free, No Harsh Preservatives**

All-Natural Ingredients

The benefits of making your own bath and body products is knowing what the ingredients are, where they came from, and allowing you peace of mind knowing that what you are putting on your skin is healthy and safe.

Small Batches

Making your own handmade bath and body products allows you to make them in smaller batches so that you are always using fresh ingredients on your skin.

Non-Toxic, Chemical & Synthetic Free, No Preservatives

By using your own all-natural ingredients you know that the product you are using is preservative free, non-toxic, chemical, and synthetic free, giving you peace of mind to enjoy your products without worry.

Vegan & Gluten Free

You can create your recipes and products using ingredients that you know are vegan and gluten free.

Cruelty Free, No Animal Testing

You know that the products that you are creating are cruelty free, and that no animal testing has been done on them, because they are coming right out of your own kitchen!

Customized

You can customize your recipes without using certain ingredients that you may know you have an allergy to, or add an ingredient that you know will help you with a particular skin problem you may have, or a scent you like the most.

Creative Packaging

The ideas for packaging have no limits. Let your

imagination soar and see what kind of interesting ideas you come up with. At a loss for ideas? Check out Pinterest.com to see what others are doing to give you inspiration!

Saves Money

The cost per patch of your own recipe using all-natural products from your own home is pennies compared to purchasing many different products at the store that serve different purposes.

Chapter 2: Basic Skincare

Skin-Care Basics

Everything you put on your skin is absorbed into your body. So why in the world are we putting nasty chemicals into and on our bodies? Let's discuss our skin for a moment.

Anatomy of the Skin

The skin is the largest organ of the body and it protects us from nasty microbes and the elements. The skin helps us to regulate our body temperature and permits sensations, such as, heat, touch, and cold.

The three layers of our skin:

- The **epidermis** is the outermost layer of our skin and provides us protection and a waterproof barrier.
- The **dermis** lays just beneath the epidermis, and contains tough connective tissue, hair follicles, and our sweat glands.
- The deepest layer is our **subcutaneous tissue** (hypodermis) and it is made of fat and connective tissue.

Skin Types

Oily Skin

If you have oily skin, you'll most obviously notice an overproduction in sebum, the clinical term for your skin's oil, but you'll also be more prone to other symptoms. Because an overproduction in oil causes pores to clog, oily skin is also commonly associated with:

- large pores
- blackheads
- blemishes
- pimples

Combination Skin

When I say combination skin, what I'm referring to is:

1. A skin type where oil is seen most commonly on forehead, nose and chin while other areas of the face are predominantly dry.
2. Skin that is affected by various skin conditions such as acne and dryness or rosacea and wrinkles.
3. Skin types that change with times of year, throughout hormonal changes or your location.

Combination skin tends to be affected by genetics, using the wrong kinds of skin care products, weather, aging and hormonal changes.

Sensitive Skin

Having sensitive skin can be frustrating, and trying new products tends to be a gamble most of us won't take. From skin care products to detergents to sunscreens, providing for your sensitive skin can be a struggle. Most commonly, those suffering from sensitive skin will experience:

- uneven skin tone
- breakouts
- rosacea
- redness
- itching
- burning
- dryness
- eczema

Acne-Prone Skin

No one is immune to acne breakouts. From puberty to hormonal changes and genetics, acne can happen to anyone. Acne is caused by hormonal changes and bacterial infections in pores, not by what you eat or how often you wash your face. Breakouts can be made worse by,touching your face, using harsh products, picking at or popping pimples, as well as using products that don't work.

Dry Skin

Dry skin can be the result of genetics or age. Dry skin can be made worse by aging,hormonal changes, weather, extended exposure to water, and products containing soaps and inadequate moisturizers. Whether you have sporadically dry skin or your skin is consistently dry, you are likely familiar with symptoms such as:

- rough and dull complexion
- reduced elasticity
- visible lines
- itchiness
- scaling

Aging Skin

As skin matures, you'll notice common and unavoidable symptoms such as:

- uneven skin tone
- lost elasticity
- sunspots
- wrinkles
- dryness

Basic Skin-Care Routine

Think of your skin-care routine as consisting of three main steps:

- **Cleansing**
- **Moisturizing**
- **Protect**

The goal of any skin-care routine is to take care of your skin so it's functioning at its best. Allow these three steps to become your daily ritual that cleanses your skin of pollutants and bacteria, Tones and balances the skin, and provides the beneficial hydration that it needs. Don't expect miraculous results overnight. Results take time.

Cleansing

The general rule of thumb here is that cleansing your complexion twice per day -- once in the morning, once in the evening -- is most preferable.

Moisturizing

Next, use a moisturizer, or a moisturizing product. It's recommend to use an oil-free, fragrance-free moisturizer.

Protect

Protecting your skin with a sunscreen can help avoid

damage from the sun and possibly avoid skin cancer. There are some sunscreens you can make yourself and you can find them later in this book.

Chapter 3: Getting Started

Note

The recipes in this book are for the home crafter and not intended for resale to the public. The cosmetic industry is a highly regulated industry and requires lengthy testing and labeling requirements to ensure safety. If you should decide to go into business selling your products it is highly advised to make sure that you're products are meeting all state and federal requirements.

If you don't know where to start you can purchase my book, **Bath & Body Business: A Girl's Guide to Starting a Homebased Business**, by Kimberly Hodge. I would also recommend that you contact your state and local government for licensing requirements. To learn more about federal requirements for small businesses and homemade cosmetics, please go here: https://www.fda.gov/cosmetics/resources-industry-cosmetics/small-businesses-homemade-cosmetics-fact-sheet

Equipment

The recipes that I have included in this book are easily created by using the equipment in your own kitchen. However, I would suggest that you keep some pots, pans, measuring cups, and spoons, separate from the items you use for cooking your meals.

Some of the equipment you will need:

- A Kitchen Scale
- Double Boiler
- Molds
- Measuring Cups
- Measuring Spoons
- Glass Bowls
- Jars and Bottles with Lids
- Stainless Steel Pans

Accurately measuring your ingredients is essential, especially if you wish to recreate your products. Having an accurate scale, measuring cups, and spoons, will help ensure that you make your products perfectly each time.

Kitchen Scale

Having a kitchen scale is an essential part of measuring ingredients for your recipes. Adding a pinch here and a pinch there without measuring is not going to be helpful for you when you go to re-create your recipe in the future.

Double Boiler

For melt and pour recipes you will need a double boiler or the use of a microwave. If you don't have a store bought double boiler you can make your own by using a larger pot for the lower chamber and a smaller pot for the upper chamber that holds your ingredients. Another idea is to use a larger pot and a heat proof container like a pyrex measuring cup, a recycled can, metal bowl, or a mason jar that is heatproof.

Measuring Cups, Spoons, Shredders

Have a good set of measuring cups and spoons that are strictly for your bath and body products. I recommend stainless steel measuring spoons and cups. Using stainless steel is more hygienic and easier to clean than plastic or wood.

I also recommend using heatproof measuring cups for heating in a microwave or to heat ingredients in. I do not recommend the use of plastic items to heat in a microwave or in boiling water. Melted plastic leaches out into your recipes and this can be toxic to you.

It is recommended to have a good shredder on hand so that you can use it to shred blocks of beeswax or soap bases.

Molds

You will need a variety of silicone molds for your lotion bar and bath bombs. You can even use ice cube trays and candy molds if your on a budget. You can purchase a variety of silicone molds and candy molds from Amazon.com. You can find a large selection of molds at a craft store as well.

Bottles and Jars

You will need an assortment of bottles and jars with lids for your various product creations.

Suggested Supplies:

- Clear Lip Balm Tubes with Lids
- BPA Free White Lip Balm Tubes with Lids
- Essential Oil Rollers
- Amber Glass Spray Bottle Atomizer
- .25 oz Metal Tins
- 1 oz Metal Tins
- 2 oz Metal Tins
- 4 oz Metal Tins
- Metal Slide Tins
- Tea Filters
- Mason Jars with Lids
- Plastic Jars and Bottles with Lids

Warning:

It's important to note that when working with oils do not store them in plastic bottles because over time they can deteriorate the plastic. The bottle with become distorted and the plastic can leach into the product.

Glass Bowls

Stocking up on a good set of glass bowls in various sizes comes in handy when mixing ingredients. You can grab some at a local department, kitchen store, or online. Personally I love the charm of a good set of country bowls that you can pick up from most antique stores or a flea market.

Stainless Pans

A good set of stainless steel pans that are strictly used for your bath and body creations is recommended. You can pick these up at your local department, kitchen store, or online.

Methods & Techniques

Making your own bath and body products requires some basic skills and creativity in the kitchen. There are a few basic methods and techniques that will be discussed in this section which will provide you the basics to making your own safe products.

Just Some Basics

The recipes in this book are suitable for beginners to make the recipes all your own. There are two heating methods you can follow.

Heating Methods

The Microwave Method

If you choose this method, make sure the containers you use are safe to use in the microwave. You'll want to start by only heating at 30 second intervals, check and stir, and then heat for an additional 10 seconds at a time to see if all the ingredients have liquefied. You want to keep your eye on the microwave to make sure you are not overheating your ingredients as the microwave cooks items quickly. Once all the items have been liquefied you can now add your botanicals, herbs, and essential oils. Pour into a container of your choice.

The Double Boiler Method

I prefer this method, however, I have at times used the microwave method. A double boiler is a pot that has a lower chamber and an upper chamber. The Upper chamber holds your ingredients and the lower holds the water that heats the ingredients without mixing with them. Put a few inches of water in the lower chamber, add your ingredients to the upper chamber, and heat until all ingredients are liquefied, using a medium heat. Once all ingredients are melted, add your botanicals, herbs, and essential oils. Pour into a container of your choice.

Techniques:

There are two techniques to making recipes in this book and they are:

- **Mix and Measure**: This is were you measure the ingredients, add the mixture into a container.

- **Melt and Pour**: In this method you measure the ingredients, melt over heat and stir, then add to a container. The melt and pour method is used in making lip balms, lotion and massage bars, and bath melts.

Both are easy to do and the results are luscious handmade products for you to use!

Warning: If you are including your children in your process you will want to provide supervision during the heating process.

Working with Preservatives

In order for your products to have any length of shelf life you will need to add a preservative. Preservatives are used in your products to stop the growth of bacteria, molds, yeast, and fungi.

You need to use preservatives when working with the following recipes:

- **Powders**

- **Water-free Products**

- **Water-based Products**

Note: Recipes to be used immediately do no not require a preservative.

Powders

Powders on first glance may appear to be waterless, however, in the case of working with clay powder it will need to be heated in an oven at 100-120 degrees Celsius or 212-248 degrees Fahrenheit for 30 minutes. This will sterilize and destroy any microbes, in addition to adding a preservative to your finished product. This powder is normally used when making facial masks.

Water-free Products

Water normally is a breeding ground for bacteria and other microorganisms. If you are making a water-free recipes, such as as oil based recipe, the a preservative is not normally required.

Water-based Products

Water-based recipes can be a breeding ground for bacteria and microorganisms, therefore, it is necessary for you to use a preservative. Using a grapefruit seed extract is safe and easy to use. It's entirely natural and a broad-spectrum antimicrobial. It's also easy to find and normally available at health food stores or online.

How to use:

The advisable amount is 1 percent of your entire recipe mixed ingredients. Increasing the dosage amount is advisable if the product you are creating has a pH of more than 7.

Always use distilled water in your recipes as it has been boiled to remove impurities, and will help your ingredients last longer.

Vitamin E Oil

Vitamin E Oil is a natural preservative that can be added into your recipes to increase shelf life. When making small batches of product at home you can purchase a small bottle of vitamin E oil capsules from the vitamin store and use two capsules per recipe.

Grapefruit Seed Extract (GSE)

A natural preservative that is used to prolong the shelf life of many bath and body products. Using a grapefruit seed extract is safe and easy to use. It's entirely natural and a broad-spectrum antimicrobial.

How to use:

The advisable amount is 1 percent of your entire recipe mixed ingredients. Increasing the dosage amount is advisable if the product you are creating has a pH of more than 7.

Citric Acid

Citric acid is a natural cleaning agent and a pH modifier. It is also a raw material manufactured specifically for industrial purposes and used in a wide variety of products, including food and beverages, pharmaceutical preparations, detergents, bath products, skincare, haircare, and many other cosmetics. Citric Acid is popular in natural formulations: it can enhance the stability and shelf-life of products, and also produce bubbles (fizzing) in desired bath or spa products. Citric Acid also has known skincare benefits and supports skin exfoliation to reveal a fresh and firmer complexion. It is also an antioxidant used in anti-aging applications.

Remember these storage and safety tips:

- Always label your products with what is in the bottle or container, ingredients, and expiration date.
- Use clean, sterilized tools, equipment, and containers.
- Never store products in direct sunlight.
- Do not leave airspace in a bottle or jar. Airspace allows for oxidation.
- Do not dip fingers into products as you can inadvertently add bacteria.
- Keep a logbook of your recipes so that you can recreate them in the future.

Expiration Dates

Review each of the ingredients that are in your individual recipes. Whichever ingredient expires first is your expiration date for your product. Recipes made with plant oils, beeswax, essential oils, and cocoa butter will last as long as the expiration of that ingredient. Recipes that include ingredients such as botanicals, sugars, herbs, and water, move up the expiration date.

Sugar is a breeding ground for bacteria and mold and should only be used for a couple of weeks then discarded. Water is also a breeding ground for bacteria and recipes including water should be used on a short term basis as well. If you notice signs of odor, discoloration, or mold, discontinue use immediately.

Using pH Strips

The pH of a substance is the measure of it's acidic or alkaline content in a water-based solution. The scale of measuring the pH balance ranges from 0-14. Neutral being 7. The further below 7 the more acidic it is, and conversely, higher than 7 the more alkaline it is.

Healthy skin is 5.5 on the scale. Most cosmetic products are formulated to be as close to the natural pH of the skin.

Any product that you are not using immediately should have a preservative added before storing. Using a grapefruit seed extract at a dosage of 1 percent in entirety to all the ingredients in your product. Grapefruit seed extract can be purchased at your local health food store or online.

When using a preservative other than grapefruit seed extract it is important to check with the manufacture of such product to determine the correct amount for your usage.

You can check the pH balance of a water-based product before adding a preservative with pH strips. These can be easily purchased online. If you are unable to obtain them online you can always check your local pet store as they are used to check the pH balance of the water in fish tanks.

Storage

Once you've created your recipes, you'll need to think about how to store your products. You need to think about how you want to package your product.

SELECTING THE RIGHT CONTAINER:

Size

Depending on the recipe you are making you may need a smaller or larger container. For example, making a lip balm of eye cream requires a smaller container than a body butter. Also, keep in mind that you do not want airspace within the jar after you add your product. This causes oxidation resulting in waste. Only make enough product for the duration that you can use before the expiration. No need to make large patches and then having to throw it away because it expired before you could use it all. This is a waste of, what could be expensive ingredients.

Pump

Recipes that contain thicker consistencies, such as creams and butters, should be placed in a jar in lieu of a pump bottle as you will not be able to pump the product through the tube. Bottles with a pump should be used for lotions, or thinner creams or gels. An atomizer pump should be used for spays, such as, toners, or perfumes.

Lids

Each container should have a secure and leak proof lid. This ensures the maximum length of shelf-life. Some lids have shive's and wad's inside the lid. This protects the products leakage.

Glass, Metal, or Plastic (New or Used?)

Using plastic containers can hold the odor of the previous product. Plastic containers are suitable for use in a shower or bath in lieu of using glass for safety reasons. For ease of use in the shower, use flip-tops or pump dispensers. As a general rule, it is recommended to use new plastic containers. If you will be re-using glass jars it is recommended that you sterilize them before each use with hot, boiling water before filling.

<u>TIPS</u>:

STORAGE

Once you purchase your ingredients, store them in airtight containers in a cool, dry place, out of sunlight. Mark the ingredients with the date of purchase.

BEFORE USE

Always check for mold, odor, and rancidity, before use of an ingredient regardless what the expiration date indicates.

AFTER CREATION

Store your products in an airtight container in the refrigerator, or a cool dry place, depending on the recipe made.

Safety

FLASH POINT

When working with oils, essential oils, and fragrance oils, it is important to check with the manufacture on it's flash point. In simplest terms possible, a fragrance oil's flash point refers to the temperature at which vapor from the oil may ignite when exposed to an open flame.

For example, if you were to heat a pot of pure fragrance oil with no wax, just oil, to the temperature listed as the fragrance oil's flash point and then light a flame at the surface of the oil where it had begun to vaporize, the vapor could potentially ignite and put you in danger of being burned.

A flash point is legally defined as "the minimum temperature at which a liquid gives off vapor within a test vessel in sufficient concentration to form an ignitable mixture with air near the surface of the liquid" under 49 CFR § 173.120 of the Code of Federal Regulations.

ESSENTIAL OILS

Many essential oils can potentially cause skin irritation. Ensure the area you are working in is well ventilated, and be sure not to get oils in your eyes. If this should happen, rinse well plenty of cold water and contact your physician.

SOURCING INGREDIENTS

Always purchase your ingredients from a trust source.

HYGIENE AND PERSONAL PROTECTIVE EQUIPMENT (PPE)

Always wear disposable vinyl gloves when measuring and handling raw ingredients. It is also advisable to wear a hairnet while making your recipes. Many wear a smock or apron when making their products for hygiene purposes as well as keeping your clothes clean from stains.

PETS

Pets do not belong in the kitchen while you are making your products.

Chapter 4: Home Apothecary

Home Apothecary

A well stocked home apothecary will be invaluable to you. Some of the ingredients you may already have in your kitchen or garden, however, if you don't have an ingredient don't fret. Many can be purchased in your local grocery, health food store, and even online. Below you will find a list of items you may want to stock in your home apothecary.

HOME APOTHECARY SUGGESTED SUPPLIES:

- Oils & Butters
- Wax
- Essential Oils
- Herbs and Flowers
- Other Supplies

Each of the above we will go through in detail.

Butters

Cocoa Butter - Is made from the cocoa bean and is an edible fat extract. It's full of antioxidants and a great choice for moisturizing the skin. Solid in its natural form, but when heated will blend nicely with other ingredients. This butter is an excellent choice for inclusion in salves, body butters, and bath melts. It is not advisable for use in facial products because it can encourage acne.

Shea Butter - This butter has a strong aroma and is better suited to be mixed with other ingredients and scented with essential oils. It has wonderful moisturizing properties for the skin and provides low level UV protection, approximately SPF-6. It contains many fatty acids that are needed to retain skin moisture and elasticity. The makes it an excellent addition to your bath and body butters.

Mango Butter - Is expeller pressed from mango seeds and is full of fatty acids, vitamins, and melts on contact with the skin. It has been used for centuries to moisturize the skin.

Essential Oils

There are a variety of quality essential oils available for use in your handcrafted bath and body products. I recommend starting with a just a few and get used to working with them before purchasing a large supply of them. The most commonly used in bath and body products are lavender, lemon, peppermint, sweet orange, and vanilla. However, I encourage you to get creative with your products. Create your own signature scent.

Essential oils are extracted from plants and is a very concentrated liquid. In many recipes you would only use a few drops of an essential oil as they are very potent.

ESSENTIAL OILS

- Basil
- Bergamot
- Cinnamon
- Ginger
- Grapefruit
- Lavender
- Lemon
- Lemongrass
- Lime
- Mandarin
- Peppermint
- Rosemary
- Spearmint

- Sweet Orange
- Vanilla

Warning:

Essential oils are very potent and can cause irritation to the skin. Do a test patch on your inner wrist and wait 24 hours to see if you have a reaction to the oil before using in your products. There are some oils that are not recommended for pregnant women to use. I highly recommend consulting a healthcare provider for approval before use. When in doubt about using essential oils, it is recommended to contact a certified aromatherapist for more information.

Herbs & Flowers

Many of the recipes in this book call for the use of dried flowers and herbs. You many use dried ingredients from your own garden, pick them up at a local natural market. You can order dried botanicals online if you can't locate them locally. Make sure when you are placing your order that you are purchasing organic, culinary grade botanicals. The following botanicals should be included in your home apothecary supplies.

BOTANICALS AND THEIR BENEFITS:

Calendula - this is golden orange in color and is very gentle and heals the skin.

Chamomile - Antibacterial, calming scent, and helps to clear up acne.

Comfrey - Reduces inflammation and incorporated into creams and lotions. Ideal for acne prone skin.

Lavender - Antibacterial properties with a soothing scent.

Mint - This has an energizing scent, and provides pain relief.

Rose - Reduces wrinkles, reduces discoloration, and increases the skin's permeability. It also provides a pink color to oils.

Sage - This is an anti-inflammatory, reduces wrinkles and reduces redness.

Oils

Olive Oil - Is the most common oil found in your kitchen making this the most convenient oil to use in your products. A rich oil with a strong aroma, yellow to green in color. If you purchase the extra virgin olive oil you will find it less aromatic making it more pleasant for skincare products. It's a stable oil and its rich consistency makes it good for conditioning the skin.

Coconut Oil - Coconut oil is known for it's benefits for the skin because of its antibacterial and antimicrobial properties. Some use pure coconut oil as a moisturizing lotion on its own and it can be combined with other oils, waxes, and butters. When purchasing a coconut oil for your handcrafted products you want to look for an unrefined virgin coconut oil.

Jojoba Oil - Made from jojoba seeds which are processed to produce a liquid wax that is similar skin absorption to our own sebum. This oil is an excellent carrier oil for use with essential oils. Jojoba oil can also be used as a cleanser.

Sweet Almond Oil - Is expressed from pressed almonds and contain fatty acids and vitamins. Sweet almond oil is a light, fragrant oil, that is popular in all-natural handcrafted beauty products recipes. This makes sweet almond oil an excellent choice for skin and hair products.

Castor Oil - This oil is made from castor beans and is unique from other oils because of it's water-binding properties allowing it to seal in moisture of the skin.

Grapeseed Oil - Is expressed from grape seeds. The oil is light and doesn't have much of an aroma. It is easily absorbed into the skin and is full of antioxidants. This oil is a great choice for facial products and is an excellent choice for those with oily skin due because of its light nature and will hydrate the skin.

Rice Bran Oil - A light oil that is vitamin-rich and is a nice addition to skincare oils, creams and lotions, protecting the skin from dryness and free radicals.

Avocado Oil - Rich in vitamin E, this oil is used for regenerative and moisturizing properties to improve the condition of hair, skin, and nails.

Argan Oil - This is a nut oil from Morocco. It is closely related to olive, but it is more difficult to harvest and is more expensive then olive oil. Argan oil is used as an anti-aging ingredient in creams, lotions, and facial oils. It has antioxidant properties and is high in vitamin E and fatty acid content.

Hemp Oil - High in essential fatty acids and is a nourishing oil for creams, lotions, and facial oils.

Wax

Beeswax - this wax is used often in bath and body products due to its ability to combine well with other ingredients and provides a more solid texture. It helps to firm balms and creams. Normally solid in solid blocks or pastilles. When choosing a beeswax for your home apothecary you would want to purchase an organic, cosmetic grade, and filtered product. The scent of filtered beeswax is much more pleasant for use in your bath and body products.

Candelilla Wax - This wax is a vegan alternative for beeswax. Can be used for lip balms, creams, balms, and lotions. It is 100% natural vegetable wax extracted from the candelilla plant.

Carnauba Wax - This wax is 100% vegan harvested from the leaves of the copernicia prunifera, commonly known as carnauba palm. Commonly used in cosmetics and personal care products such as, lip balms, balms, ointments, and deodorant.

Other Supplies

In addition to the previously mentioned supplies for your home apothecary, there are other ingredients and supplies you may want to have on hand. Many of the items you may already have in your kitchen cupboard or bathroom cabinet.

It is recommended that you purchase the purest, all-natural, and organic ingredients so that you are handcrafting a safe and healthy product for yourself and others. The items recommended here can be found in your local grocery, health food stores, and online.

Purchasing from a specialist online supplier will provide you consistant, quality ingredients from a company you can trust. Contact the supplier and ask questions regarding their product sourcing, production process, product storage, and shipping procedures.

Having answers to these important questions will give you peace of mind, provide you knowledge to your customers, and help you answer questions when your customers ask you how you source your ingredients.

Aloe Vera Gel

Aloe vera gel is known for its anti-inflammatory, skin soothing, and moisturizing properties. Pick up a quality gel at a local health food store. Aloe can help soothe sunburns with a natural cooling effect.

Chia Seeds

Chia seeds are rich in omega-3 fatty acids. They are great for nourishing and exfoliating the skin. You can add these to soaps and scrubs.

Coffee Beans

When added to a soap bar or a body scrub, finely ground coffee beans can rid the skin of dry, dead skin cells and restore it to a more radiant and smooth appearance. Coffee, by stimulating blood flow, improves circulation and consequently the appearance of the skin.

Dried Milk Powder

Dried milk powder can be added into creams, lotions, and bath soaks.

Glycerin

Vegetable glycerin naturally attracts moisture when applied to the skin.

Goat Milk Powder

It possesses anti-inflammatory properties and can help reduce the effects of skin conditions such as psoriasis, eczema and rosacea. The benefits of using goats milk outweighs the use of harsh chemicals used in normal soaps, and goat milk lotions, creams and soaps are far better for your skin that normal skin cleansers. It is rich in nutrients, a natural exfoliant, and may prevent acne. **Dried goat milk powder can be added into creams,** lotions, and bath soaks.

Manuka Honey

Manuka honey is produced only in New Zealand by bees pollinating the native manuka bush. This honey is known for its anti-inflammatory and healing properties.

Kaolin (White Clay)

This a base for face masks on account for its ability to absorb impurities and toxins from the skin.

Natural Colorants

You want your products to be all-natural and organic as possible and therefore you should use natural colorants in your recipes. The following natural ingredients should be a part of your home apothecary.

<u>Natural Colorants:</u>

Brown - Use cocoa powder.
Green - Use spirulina or sage powder.
Golden-Yellow - Use safflower powder.
Orange - for a yellowish orange use annatto seed powder, and for a reddish orange use paprika.
Pink - Use madder root or beet root powder.
Purple - Use ratanjot powder.
Yellow - Use tumeric.

Natural Soap

Grated un-perfumed soap is often used as a cleaning ingredient in bath and foot powders.

Oatmeal

Organic oatmeal can be ground down into a fine powder and used in face masks as a gentle exfoliator. You can use whole or coursely ground oatmeal in soaps as well to provide an exfoliating aspect.

Oat Bran & Rice Bran Powder

This will provide a course-textured powdered ingredient to facial scrubs and and bath soaks.

Oranges & Lemons

Fresh lemon juice can be used in hair rinse, and the zest of lemons and oranges can be used in exfoliating hand scrubs.

Salts

Salt helps to exfoliate the skin while naturally detoxifying. It contains a high level of naturally occurring minerals and is both detoxifying and exfoliating to the skin. It is also known to heal minor skin conditions. Salt can be added to baths, or used in bath and body hand scrubs. Epsom salt helps to soothe aching muscles when added to a bath.

There are a few salts to choose from:

- Sea Salt
- Epsom Salt
- Pink Himalayan Sea Salt

Sodium Bicarbonate (Baking Soda)

It is an essential ingredient in making bath bombs, and fizzy bath powders when combining baking soda.

Witch Hazel

Witch hazel soothes irritated skin, including acne. It can tighten and moisture the skin as well.

Chapter 5: Skincare Recipes

Body

In this section you will find a recipes for calming, moisturizing, soothing, energizing, and more!

<h1 align="center">Balms & Butters</h1>

Butters

{Sore Muscle Butter}

Ingredients:

1/2 cup coconut oil
1/2 cup shea butter
10 drops peppermint essential oil
15 drops tea tree essential oil

Directions:

Mix shea butter and coconut oil into a microwave safe mixing bowl. Microwave in 30 second increment at 50 percent power. Stir until mixture liquefies. Remove bowl with an oven mitt and stir until clear.

Turn the mixture into cream by covering the bowl with plastic wrap and let cool in the refrigerator until the texture resembles softened butter. If mixture fully hardens, remove from refrigerator and let it warm on the counter. Add essential oil, then whip with a hand mixture on low speed for 3-5 minutes, or until the color brightens and peaks form in the mixture.

When desired consistency is reached, scoop into a jar with spatula. Makes about 1 cup. Store in a cool, dry place. Use within 3-4 weeks.

Whipped Body Butter

{Cinnamon Vanilla Whipped Body Butter}

Ingredients:

1/2 cup shea butter
1/4 cup coconut oil
1/2 tbsp jojoba oil
1/2 tsp ground cinnamon
1/2 tsp vanilla extract

Directions:

Mix shea butter and coconut oil into a microwave safe mixing bowl. Microwave in 30 second increment at 50 percent power. Stir until mixture liquefies. Remove bowl with an oven mitt and stir until clear.

Turn the mixture into cream by covering the bowl with plastic wrap and let cool in the refrigerator until the texture resembles softened butter. If mixture fully hardens, remove from refrigerator and let it warm on the counter. Add cinnamon and vanilla, then whip with a hand mixer on low speed for 3-5 minutes or until the color brightens and peaks form.

When desired consistency is reached, scoop into a jar with spatula. Makes about 1 cup. Store in a cool, dry place. Use within 3-4 weeks.

Bath

Bath Bombs

{Fizzy Bath Bomb}

Ingredients:

2 cups baking soda
1 cup citric acid
100% pure witch hazel
Spray Bottle
10-20 drops of essential oils of your choice
Natural Colorant (optional)
Plastic Mold

Directions:

In a large mixing bowl, measure in the baking soda, citric acid, and mix well. Add a 1/2 tsp of coloring and mix well. The color will become more pronounced when you add more witch hazel. Keep in mind that the more colorant used it may leave a ring around the tub. Add 20-30 drops of essential oils and mix well. Using an atomizer or spray bottle filled with witch hazel, lightly spray the entire surface of the powder and mix with your hands at the same time. Keep spraying and mixing rapidly until the mixture holds together when scrunched with your hand. Be careful not to add too much witch hazel - a little goes a long way.

Working quickly, firmly press mixture into molds. Use molds large enough for the bath bomb to combine and set. To make a round bath bomb, fill both sides of the mold and press them together firmly. Tap gently to release the bath bomb from the mold. Let dry for 30 minutes or until they don't fall apart.

To Use:

Drop into a warm water bath and enjoy!

Bath Melts

{Bathing Beauty Melts}

Ingredients:

1 cup shea butter
1 tbsp coconut oil
2 tbsp epsom salt
1/4 cup baking soda
10 drops lavender essential oil (optional)
5 drops roman chamomile essential oil (optional)
1 tbsp pink edible shimmer dust (optional)
Silicone molds

Directions:

Mix shea butter and coconut oil into a microwave safe mixing bowl. Microwave in 30 second increment at 50 percent power. Stir until mixture liquefies. Remove bowl with an oven mitt and stir until clear. Stir in coconut oil until melted.

Stir in epsom salts, baking soda, essential oils, and shimmer dust. Pour mixture into silicone treat molds and let harden at room temperature. Makes five or six medium sized bath melts. Store individually in a cool, dry place.

To Use:

To use just drop into your tub and enjoy a spa like

experience.

Bath Salts

{Lavender Bath Salts}

Ingredients:

1 cup sea salt
1 cup epsom salt
10 drops lavender essential oil
2-3 drops purple food coloring (optional)

Directions:

Pour salts into a lidded glass container. Add essential oil, then add food coloring. Stir all ingredients together. Makes 2 cups or enough for two soaks. Store extra for up to two weeks in a cool, dry place.

{Peppermint Bath Salts}

Ingredients:

1 cup sea salt
1 cup epsom salt
10 drops peppermint essential oil
2-3 drops green food coloring (optional)

Directions:

Pour salts into a lidded glass container. Add essential oil, then add food coloring. Stir all ingredients together. Makes 2 cups or enough for two soaks. Store extra for up to two weeks in a cool, dry place.

To Use:

Dissolve bath salts into warm water, then soak inside the tub for 20 minutes to enjoy the detoxifying benefits.

{Botanical Test Tube Bath Salts}

Recipe #1 - Lavender

Ingredients:

3/8 cup of Epsom Salt
1/4 cup of dried Lavender buds
10 drops of Lavender essential oils

Directions:

Mix ingredients in a bowl and pour into a 85 gram glass test tube with lid or cork. Use caution with glass around bathtub.

Recipe #2 - Rose

Ingredients:

3/8 cup of Epsom Salt
1/4 cup of dried Rose petals
10 drops of Rose essential oils

Directions:

Mix ingredients in a bowl and pour into a 85 gram glass test tube with lid or cork. Use caution with glass around bathtub.

Recipe #3 - Citrus

Ingredients:

3/8 cup of Empsom Salt
1/4 cup of dried Citrus and Zest
10   drops Citrus essential oil blend or any combination of grapefruit, lime, lemon, sweet orange, tangerine, and bergamot.

Directions:

Mix ingredients in a bowl and pour into a 85 gram glass test tube with lid or cork. Use caution with glass around bathtub.

Bath Soaps

Melt and pour soaps recipes are the best option for new soap creators. They are the easiest to learn and the safest to work with.

Here are two excellent resources to learn the soap making process:

Soap Queen by Brambleberry -

https://www.soapqueen.com/

Wholesale Supplies Plus Soap Making -

Http://www.wholesalesuppliesplus.com/handmade101/how-to-make-recipes/melt-and-pour-soap-making.aspx

{Goats Milk Melt & Pour Soap}

Ingredients:

2 cups of melt and pour organic goat milk soap base cut into cubes so they melt faster
3 tbsp of organic jojoba oil or organic almond oil
Himalayan Salts
20 Drops of Sweet Orange Essential Oil
5 Drops of All Spice Essential Oil
10 Drops of Frankincense Essential Oils (or any essential oils of your choice - total max 30 drops)

Directions:

Step 1: Chop soap base into cubes.

Step 2: Add them to your double boiler on low to medium heat.

Step 3: Continue stirring until the soap bas is melted.

Step 4: Once Melted, add the jojoba or almond oil, mix well. You could also substitute with any carrier oil of your choice.

Step 5: Add essential oils if desired, mix well.

Step 6: Sprinkle a little bit of Himalayan Salt at the bottom of the mold.

Step 7: Pour into the silicone mold.

Step 8: Spray pure alcohol on the top of the soap to get rid of the bubbles if any.

Step 9: Add the Himalayan Salt on the top of the soaps while the soap is still liquid.

Step 10: Let dry for 24 hours before removing from mold.

{Lemon Goats Milk Melt & Pour Soap}

Ingredients:

28 oz. Goat Milk melt and pour base

10 mL Lemon Essential Oil
1.5 tsp Lemon Peel
Yellow Oxide Color Block
99% Isopropyl Alcohol

Directions:

Step 1: Chop and melt 2 oz. of Goat Milk melt and pour base in the microwave using 10 second bursts. Do this until its completely melted. Don't over cook it or it will scorch.

Step 2: Add shavings of the Yellow Oxide color block until a rich yellow color is achieved. Dispersing the powder helps avoid clumps.

Step 3: Once melted, add 10 mL of Lemon Essential Oil and use a spoon or spatula to fully mix in.

Step 4: Once the soap has reached a temperature of 120-125 degrees Fahrenheit, pour soap into the mold, and spritz the top with 99% alcohol to disperse any bubbles.

Step 5: Allow to fully cool and harden.

Step 6: Once cooled and hardened, remove from the mold and use a sharp knife to cut into bars along the score lines if using a loaf mold or pop out of the individual silicone molds.

Tub Teas

{Calming Tub Tea}

Ingredients:

3 x 4 inch organza bag
1/2 cup oats
1/2 cup powdered milk
1/4 cup epsom salts
1 tsp baking soda

Directions:

Blend oats in a food processor or blender. Mix all ingredients in a bowl with a pour spout, then stir. Pour into organza bag and tie in a knot. Makes one bag.

{Re-energizing Tub Tea}

Ingredients:

3 x 4 inch organza bag
1/2 cup oats
1/2 cup epsom salts
1/4 cup course sea salt
5 drops peppermint essential oil
10 drops lemon essential oil
10 drops orange essential oil

Directions:

Blend oats in a food processor or blender. Mix all ingredients in a bowl with a pour spout, then stir. Pour into organza bag and tie in a knot. Makes one bag.

To Store:

Store organza bag in a reusable zip-lock bag until needed.

To Use:

Fill bathtub with warm water, place organza bag directly in the water and let soak for the duration of your bath.

Salt Scrubs

Scrubs

{Mocha Salt Scrub}

Ingredients:

1/2 cup course sea salt
1/4 cup ground coffee
1/4 cup olive oil
1 tbsp cocoa powder
1/2 tsp vanilla extract

Directions:

Mix all ingredients in a bowl. Stir together, then scoop into a lidded jar. Makes about 1 cup. Store in a cool, dry place.

To Use:

Dissolve bath salts into warm water, then soak inside the tub for 20 minutes. The salts in this recipe have detoxifying benefits.

{Healing Himalayan Pink Salt Scrub}

Ingredients:

1 cup of Pink Himalayan Sea Salt
1/2 cup of Coconut Oil
1/3 cup of Rose-infused Sweet Almond Oil
8 drops of Rose Geranium essential Oil
Dried Rose petals

Directions:

Mix all ingredients in a bowl. Stir together, then scoop into a lidded, airtight container. Store in a cool, dry place.

To Use:

Dissolve bath salts into warm water, then soak inside the tub for 20 minutes. The salts in this recipe have detoxifying benefits.

Shower Scrub

{Vanilla Honey Scrub}

Ingredients:

1 cup white sugar
1/4 cup olive oil
2 tbsp honey
1/2 tsp vanilla extract

Directions:

Mix all ingredients in a small bowl. Store in a lidded glass container. Makes about 1 cup. Store in a cool, dry place.

To Use:

Massage a small handful onto your body and rinse while in the shower.

{Peppermint Coconut Sugar Scrub}

Ingredients:

1 Cup of Sugar
5/8 cup of Virgin Coconut Oil
1 Mint Tea Bag
10 Drops of Peppermint essential oil
1/4 tsp of Spirulina powder (optional)

Directions:

Mix all ingredients in a small bowl. Store in a lidded glass container. Makes about 1 cup. Store in a cool, dry place.

To Use:

Massage a small handful onto your body and rinse off while in the shower.

Shower Steamers

Note: Use gloves when making these recipes as citric acid can irritate the skin.

{Calming Shower Steamer}

Ingredients:

1 cup of baking soda
1/2 cup citric acid
1 tbsp witch hazel in a spray bottle
5 drops lavender essential oil
10 drops roman chamomile essential oil
5 drops orange essential oil
Silicone mold
Rubber gloves

Directions:

In a large bowl, combine the baking soda and citric acid. Stir until smooth and all lumps are removed. Add essential oils and stir. Spritz mixture with 5-10 sprays of witch hazel, then mix with your hands (use gloves).

Continue until mixture is slightly damp, but not wet enough to form a ball. Use as little witch hazel as possible, otherwise the shower steamers will expand as they dry.

When the mixture reaches the desired texture, press it

firmly into silicone molds. Let dry overnight. Remove carefully from the molds, then store in a resealable plastic bag or glass jar. Makes about 5 small shower steamers.

To Use:

Wet a steamer in your shower, place on the side of the tub.

{Energizing Shower Steamer}

Ingredients:

1 cup baking soda
1/2 cup citric acid
1 tbsp witch hazel in spray bottle
5 drops peppermint essential oil
10 drops lemon essential oil
10 drops orange essential oil
Silicone mold
Rubber gloves

Directions:

In a large bowl, combine the baking soda and citric acid. Stir until smooth and all lumps are removed. Add essential oils and stir. Spritz mixture with 5-10 sprays of witch hazel, then mix with your hands (use gloves).

Continue until mixture is slightly damp, but not wet enough to form a ball. Use as little witch hazel as possible, otherwise the shower steamers will expand as they dry.

When the mixture reaches the desired texture, press it firmly into silicone molds. Let dry overnight. Remove carefully from the molds, then store in a resealable plastic bag or glass jar.

Makes about 5 small shower steamers.

To Use:

Wet a steamer in your shower, place on the side of the tub.

Creams & Lotions

Creams

{Sweet Dreams Cream}

Ingredients:

1 cup coconut oil
15 drops lavender essential oil
25 drops roman chamomile essential oil

Directions:

Scoop the coconut oil into a mixing bowl. Consistency should be that of soften butter. Add essential oil, then whip with a hand mixer on low speed for 3-5 minutes or until the color brightens and peaks form.

When desired consistency is reached, scoop into a jar with a spatula. Depending on how much the ingredients are whipped, this recipe makes about enough to fill a 4 ounce jar. Store in a cool, dry place.

To Use:

Massage this salve on your hands, feet, and temples.

Lotion Bars

{Luxurious Lotion Bars}

Ingredients:

1/2 cup coconut oil
1/2 cup shea butter
1/2 cup grated beeswax or beeswax pastilles
20 drops roman chamomile essential oil
Silicone mold

Directions:

Mix shea butter and beeswax into a microwave safe bowl with a pour spout. Microwave in 30 second increments at 50 percent power, stirring each time, until mixture becomes liquid. Remove bowl with an oven mitt. Stir in coconut oil until clear, not cloudy. Let cool slightly, then add essential oil.

Using an oven mitt, carefully pour liquid into silicone molds. Let harden overnight at room temperature, then remove carefully from mold. Store in an a airtight container in a cool, dry place.

To Use:

The warmth of your hands will melt these luxurious creamy bars allowing you to massage into your hands, arms, legs, and feet.

Feet

{Foot Repair Stick}

Ingredients:

1/3 cup of coconut oil
1/3 cup grated beeswax or beeswax pastilles
3 tbsp shea butter
16 drops tea tree essential oil (optional)
Empty Deodorant tube

Directions:

Mix shea butter and beeswax into a microwave safe bowl with a pour spout. Microwave in 30 second increments at 50 percent power, stirring each time, until mixture liquefies. Remove bowl from microwave with an oven mitt. Stir in coconut oil until clear, not cloudy. Let cool slightly, then add essential oil.

Create a tight seal at the bottom of an empty deodorant tube by screwing canister to its lowest setting. If you would like to buy a new deodorant tube please see resource section. Place cap on the top of tube and keep in the refrigerator overnight until liquid solidifies.

Makes enough to fill an empty deodorant tube. Store in a cool, dry place. Use within 3-4 weeks.

To Use:

Use this stick on the heels of your feet before bed, slip on a a warm pair of socks then enjoy soft, smooth feet in the morning!

Foot Scrub

{Gingerbread Foot Scrub}

Ingredients:

1/2 cup packed brown sugar
1/2 cup white sugar
3 tbsp olive oil
1/2 tsp ground ginger
1/4 tsp ground cinnamon
1/4 tsp allspice
1/4 tsp nutmeg
1/2 tsp vanilla extract

Directions:

Mix all ingredients in a small bowl. Scoop into a lidded glass container. Makes about 1 cup. Store in a cool, dry place, and use within 3-4 weeks.

To Use:

Massage a handful onto your feet while sitting over a bathtub or a large bowl of water with a towel underneath.

{Tingly Salt Scrub}

Ingredients:

1 cup sea salt
1/2 cup olive oil
12 drops peppermint essential oil

12 drops tea tree essential oil

Directions:

Mix all ingredients in a small bowl. Place mixture in a lidded glass container. Makes about 1 cup. Store in a cool, dry place. Use within 3-4 weeks.

To Use:

Massage a handful onto your feet while sitting over a bathtub or a large bowl of water with a towel underneath.

Foot Soaks

{Soothing Soak}

Ingredients:

1 cup powdered milk
1/2 cup epsom salts
5 drops lavender essential oil (optional)
3 drops orange essential oil (optional)

Directions:

Mix all ingredients in a bowl, then pour into a lidded glass container until ready to use. Each recipe makes 1 1/2 cups, or enough for two foot soaks.

{Re-Energizing Mix}

Ingredients:

1 cup baking soda
1/2 cup epsom salts
10 drops peppermint essential oil

Directions:

Mix all ingredients in a bowl, then pour into a lidded glass container until ready to use. Each recipe makes 1 1/2 cups, or enough for two foot soaks.

To Use:

Fill a large bowl big enough for both feet. I plastic dish pan is an excellent choice for this soak. Fill halfway with warm water.

Pour 3/4 cup of the mix into the bowl. Soak your feet for 10-15 minutes, then pat dry with a clean towel. Discard the remaining liquid down the toilet and flush away!

Foot Spray

{Fresh Foot Spray}

Ingredients:

4 tbsp apple cider vinegar
2 tbsp distilled water
6 drops tea tree essential oil

Directions:

Mix all ingredients in a small bowl with a pour spout. Pour into a 3 ounce spray bottle. Store in a cool, dry place. Use within 2 weeks.

To Use:

Spritz this on your feet to absorb smells. Tea tree oil helps to tame toenail fungus, and its deodorizing and healing as well!

Hands

Cuticle Balm

{Lavender Balm}

Ingredients:

6 tsp shea butter
3 tsp grated beeswax or beeswax pastilles
3 tsp jojoba oil
3 drops lavender essential oil

Directions:

Mix shea butter and beeswax into a microwave-safe bowl. Use a glass measuring cup with a pour spout. Microwave in 30 seconds increments at 50% power then stir. When fully liquid, remove with an oven mitt and stir. Add jojoba oil and stir. Let cool then add essential oil. Pour ingredients into small containers that have a lid. Let harden at room temperature. Recipe makes enough for six small round tin containers. Store in a cool dry place. Use within 3-4 weeks.

To Use:

Massage on and around your nails three times per week.

{Lemon Balm}

Ingredients:

6 tsp shea butter
3 tsp grated beeswax or beeswax pastilles
3 tsp jojoba oil
3 drops lemon essential oil

Directions:

Mix shea butter and beeswax into a microwave-safe bowl. Use a glass measuring cup with a pour spout. Microwave in 30 seconds increments at 50% power then stir. When fully liquid, remove with an oven mitt and stir. Add jojoba oil and stir. Let cool then add essential oil. Pour ingredients into small containers that have a lid. Let harden at room temperature. Recipe makes enough for six small round tin containers. Store in a cool dry place. Use within 3-4 weeks.

To Use:

Massage on and around your nails three times per week.

Hand Cream

{Lavender Hand Cream}

Ingredients:

1/4 Cup shea butter
1 tbsp beeswax or beeswax pastilles
1/8 cup jojoba oil
6 drops lavender essential oil

Directions:

Mix shea butter and beeswax into a microwave-safe bowl. Use a glass measuring cup with a pour spout. Microwave in 30 seconds increments at 50% power then stir. When fully liquid, remove with an oven mitt and stir. Add jojoba oil and stir. Let cool then add essential oil. Carefully pour mixture into lidded glass jar. Let solidify at room temperature overnight. Makes about 1/2 cup or enough to fill a 4-ounce glass container. Store in a cool dry place. Use within 3-4 weeks.

To Use:

Massage a small amount into your hands, then pat dry with a dry paper towel.

Hand Scrub

{Energizing Citrus Scrub}

Ingredients:

1 cup sea salt
1/2 cup olive oil
15-20 drops lemon or orange oil

Directions:

Mix all ingredients in a bowl. Scoop into a lidded glass container. Makes about 1 cup. Stir before each use. Store in a cool, dry place. Use within 3-4 weeks.

To Use:

Use a small amount into your hands, massage over the sink, rinse, then pat dry.

{Antibacterial Hand Scrub}

Ingredients:

1 cup sea salt
1/2 cup olive oil
15-20 drops of tea tree essential oil

Directions:

Mix all ingredients in a bowl. Scoop into a lidded glass container. Makes about 1 cup. Stir before each use. Store in a cool, dry place. Use within 3-4 weeks.

To Use:

Use a small amount into your hands, massage over the sink, rinse, then pat dry.

Nail Serum

{Nail Strengthening Serum}

Ingredients:

4 tbsp jojoba oil
2 tbsp olive oil
10 drops lavender essential oil
5 drops lemon essential oil

Directions:

Mix all ingredients together in a bowl with a pour spout. Pour into a glass bottle that has a dropper. Makes enough to fill a 3-ounce bottle. Store in a cool, dry place. Use within 3-4 weeks.

To Use:

Add one drop to each nail. Massage into each nail and cuticle. Apply three times a week until your nails feel moisturized.

Hair

Shampoo

{Dry Shampoo}

Ingredients:

1/4 cup cornstarch
1 tbsp baking soda
2 drops lavender essential oil

Directions:

Combine ingredients in a bowl and stir. Scoop into a container. Makes enough to fill a 3 ounce spice jar.

To Use:

Use when you don't have time to wash your hair and it needs a pick me up. Sprinkle a little of this powder into your hair in the greasy areas, tassel and go.

{Coconut Milk - Ylang Shampoo}

Ingredients:

3/4 cup liquid castile soap
1/2 cup canned coconut milk
1 tbsp coconut oil
15 drops Ylang Ylang essential oil

Directions:

Step 1: In a medium bowl, whisk together the castile soap,

coconut milk, and coconut oil until blended. This should take about a minute.

Step 2: Whisk in the Ylang Ylang essential oil and pour the shampoo into a jar or bottle with a lid.

Step 3: Store the shampoo for up to 1 month. Shake before using.

Conditioner

{Deep Conditioning Treatment}

Ingredients:

6 tbsp coconut oil
4 tbsp shea butter
2 tsp jojoba oil

Directions:

Scoop shea butter into a microwave safe bowl with a pour spout. Microwave in 30 second increments at 50 percent power, Stirring each time, until it becomes liquid. Remove bowl with an oven mitt. Stir in coconut oil until mixture is clear. Add jojoba oil and stir. Pour into a 4 ounce jar. Let sit overnight so oils and butter can cool to form a cream.

To Use:

Massage a small amount in to damp hair. Leave in for 10 minutes then shampoo and rinse.

Hair Mask

{No More Frizz Mask}

Ingredients:

1 ripe banana
1/4 cup plain yogurt, or more for longer hair
1 tbsp honey

Directions:

Put banana and yogurt in a bowl and mix and mash together with a fork. Add honey and stir until blended well. Makes one mask.

To Use:

Evenly apply to hair then wrap hair with plastic wrap or shower cap. Leave mask in for 10 minutes, then rinse. Shampoo and condition as normal.

{Deep Conditioning Mask}

Ingredients:

1/2 ripe avocado
1/4 cup mayonnaise, or more for long hair
1 tbsp olive oil

Directions:

Put avocado and mayonnaise in a bowl and mix and mash together with a fork. Add olive oil and stir until blended well.

Makes one mask.

To Use:

Evenly apply to hair then wrap hair with plastic wrap or shower cap. Leave mask in for 10 minutes, then rinse. Shampoo and condition as normal.

Face

Face Creams

{Light Shea Butter Face Cream}

This recipe is light enough to be used underneath makeup and suitable for most skin types.

Ingredients:

Phase 1

1/2 tsp glycerine
4 3/4 tbsp orange flower water
2 tsp sweet almond oil
1 1/2 tsp *olivem 1000
1 tsp shea butter
1/2 tsp vitamin E oil in dilution

Phase 2

1/2 tsp evening primrose oil
5 drops neroli essential oil in dilution
20 drops grapefruit seed extract as a preservative

Directions:

Measure the glycerine, orange flower water, sweet almond oil, olivem 1000, shea butter and vitamin E oil into a heatproof measuring cup or bowl with a pour spout. Heat heatproof container in double boiler until all ingredients have melted completely about 158-176 degrees. Maintain the temperature for 30 minutes. Remove from heat with an oven mitt. Whip the mixture with a hand mixer. Cool to 104 degrees in a water bath, add phase 2 ingredients and stir into a sterilized, airtight jar or container. Label with the date and ingredients used.

To Use:

Apply to clean dry face. Gently massage a small amount onto face and neck areas.

NOTE: Olivem 1000 is naturally derived from olive oil with a mix of Cetearyl (emulsion stabilizer) and Sorbitan (sorbitol). Its best used for making oil-in-water emulsions (creams where the oil is the internal/dispersed phase and the water phase is more than 45%).

Makes: About 3 1/2 ounces

{Shea Butter Night Cream}

This is a rich cream with a thoroughly indulgent feel.

Ingredients:

1 tsp glycerine
4 tbsp rose water
2 tsp grapeseed oil
1/4 oz shea butter
1/4 tsp beeswax white BP
6 drops jasmine essential oil in dilution
20 drops grapefruit seed extract as a preservative

Directions:

Measure all the ingredients apart from the jasmine oil and preservative into a heatproof bowl with spout or measuring cup. Follow the method of preparation for the light shea butter face cream. After mixture has cooled to 104 degrees, add the jasmine oil and preservative. Stir and mix thoroughly and pour into a sterilized, airtight jar. Label with the date and ingredients used.

To Use:

Apply to clean dry face. Gently massage a small amount onto face and neck areas.

Makes: About 3 1/2 ounces

Facial Refresher Spray

{Refreshing Facial Spray}

Ingredients:

1/4 cup aloe vera gel
5 drops peppermint essential oil
1/4 tsp witch hazel

Directions:

Mix all ingredients in a bowl with a pour spout. Pour into a 2 ounce spray bottle.

To Use:

Shake before use, avoid contact with your eyes by covering them with your hand or a washcloth. Store in the refrigerator to keep spray extra cool.

Facial Wash

{Warming Lemon Honey Face Wash}

Ingredients:

3 tbsp honey
3 tbsp vegetable glycerin
3 drops lemon essential oil

Directions:

Stir all ingredients in a bowl with a pour spout. Pour into a plastic squeeze bottle or tube. This recipe makes enough to fill a 3 ounce bottle.

To Use:

Gently massage a small amount in circular motions onto your dry face. It will warm naturally as your rub into your skin. Pat dry and clean with a towel.

Note: Look for raw unrefined honey in lieu of processed honey. It is more beneficial for your skin.

Moisturizers

{Calming Face Lotion}

Ingredients:

1/4 cup shea butter
4 tbsp jojoba oil
10-15 drops lavender essential oil

Directions:

Put shea butter into a microwavable mixing bowl. Microwave in 30 second increments at 50 percent power, stirring each time, until it becomes liquid. Remove bowl with an oven mitt and stir until clear, not cloudy. Add jojoba oil and stir.

To turn the liquid into a cream, cover the bowel the plastic wrap and place in the refrigerator until the texture resembles softened butter this step should take no longer than an hour. Add essential oil, then whip with a hand mixer on low speed for 3-5 minutes or until the color brightens and peaks form.

When desired consistency is reached, scoop into a lidded glass jar with a spatula. Makes about 1/2 cup.

To Use:

Massage a small amount onto your face and neck. Remember you only need a small amount.

{Acne-Fighting Face Lotion}

Ingredients:

1/4 cup shea butter
4 tbsp jojoba oil
1-15 drops tea tree essential oil

Directions:

Put shea butter into a microwavable mixing bowl. Microwave in 30 second increments at 50 percent power, stirring each time, until it becomes liquid. Remove bowl with an oven mitt and stir until clear, not cloudy. Add jojoba oil and stir.

To turn the liquid into a cream, cover the bowel the plastic wrap and place in the refrigerator until the texture resembles softened butter this step should take no longer than an hour. Add essential oil, then whip with a hand mixer on low speed for 3-5 minutes or until the color brightens and peaks form.

When desired consistency is reached, scoop into a lidded glass jar with a spatula. Makes about 1/2 cup.

To Use:

Massage a small amount onto your face and neck. Remember you only need a small amount.

Sprays

{Skin-Soothing Spray}

Ingredients:

2 tbsp aloe vera gel
4 tbsp rosewater
3 drops roman chamomile essential oil (optional)

Directions:

Mix all ingredients in a bowl with a pour spout. Pour into a glass spray bottle. This recipe makes enough to fill a 2 ounce spray bottle.

To Use:

Shake before each use. Avoid contact with your eyes by covering with a wash rag or hold your hand over your eyes.

Toners

{Rosewater Toner}

Ingredients:

1/4 cup rosewater
2 tbsp witch hazel
1/4 tsp vegetable glycerin

Directions:

Mix ingredients in a bowl with a pour spout. Pour mixture into a lidded container. Makes enough to fill a 3 ounce bottle.

To Use:

First clean your face, then apply a toner with a cotton ball. Shake before each use, and avoid contact with your eyes.

Face Masks

{Chocolate Mousse Face Mask}

Ingredients:

1 tbsp honey
2 tsp cocoa powder
1 tsp jojoba oil or olive oil
1/4 tsp fine sea salt

Directions:

Mix all ingredients together in a bowl. Stir until mixture forms a pudding like paste. This recipe makes one mask.

To Use: Gently massage a thin layer onto face, avoid the eye area. Leave on for 10 minutes, then rinse off mask completely before patting face dry with a clean towel.

NOTE: If face mask stings wash it off your skin immediately.

{Good Morning Face Mask}

Ingredients:

1 tsp powdered milk
1 tsp honey
3 tsp plain yogurt

Directions:

Mix all ingredients together in a bowl. Stir until mixture

forms a pudding like paste. This recipe makes one mask.

To Use: Gently massage a thin layer onto face, avoid the eye area. Leave on for 10 minutes, then rinse off mask completely before patting face dry with a clean towel.

NOTE: If face mask stings wash it off your skin immediately.

Scrubs

{Exfoliating Face Scrub}

Ingredients:

3 tsp baking soda
2 tsp jojoba oil

Directions:

Mix all ingredients in a small bowl. This recipe makes enough for a single use.

To Use:

Gently massage a small amount in circular motions onto your dry face. Rinse with warm water, then pat with a clean towel.

Lip Care

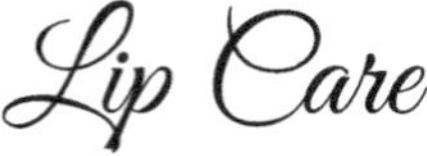

{Coconut Lip Balm}

Ingredients:

2 tbsp coconut oil
2 tbsp grated beeswax or beeswax pastilles
4 tsp olive oil

Directions:

Scoop beeswax and coconut oil into a microwave safe bowl with pour spot. Microwave in 30 second increments at 50 percent power, stirring each time, until the mixture becomes liquid. Remove bowl with an oven mitt and stir until clear. Add olive oil and stir.

Carefully pour into small, clear, circular storage containers with screw-top lids. Let harden at room temperature, then screw on caps. This recipe makes about six lip balms.

To Use:

Apply to your lips to enjoy luxurious moisturizing.

{Candy Cane Lip Balm}

Ingredients:

4 tbsp castor oil
4 tsp beeswax pastilles
1 tsp carnauba wax
16 drops peppermint essential oil
10 drops vanilla essential oil

Directions:

Melt oil and waxes in a double boiler. Remove from heat and add essential oils, blend well. Pour into tubes and leave untouched until cool and solidified.

To Use:

Apply to your lips to enjoy!

Lip Scrub

{Vanilla Coffee Lip Scrub}

Ingredients:

1/4 cup sugar
1 tsp ground coffee
1 tbsp olive oil
1 tsp vanilla extract

Directions:

Mix the ingredients together in a small bowel. Scoop a portion into a small, clear, circular storage container with a screw lid. This recipe makes about five portions.

To Use:

Use your finger to scoop out a small amount then rub onto your lips in a circular motion. Rinse off excess.

Miscellaneous Recipes

Bug Be Gone

{Bug Be Gone Spray}

Ingredients:

3 tbsp witch hazel
2 tbsp distilled water
1/2 tsp vegetable glycerin
15 drops tea tree essential oil
5 drops lavender essential oil

Directions:

Mix ingredients in a glass bowl with a pour spout. Pour into a 2 ounce spray bottle.

To Use:

Spritz on exposed skin avoiding contact with eyes.

Deodorant

{Deodorant For Sensitive Skin}

Ingredients:

1/3 cup coconut oil
1/3 cup grated beeswax or beeswax pastilles
1/3 cup cornstarch
3 tbsp shea butter
2 tbsp baking soda
15 drops tea tree essential oil

Directions:

Mix beeswax and shea butter into a microwave safe bowl with pour spout. Microwave in 30 second increments at 50 percent power, stirring each time, until it mostly liquid. Remove bowl with an oven mitt. Stir in coconut oil until clear, not cloudy. Let cool slightly, then stir in additional ingredients.

Create a tight seal at the bottom of an empty deodorant tube by screwing canister to its lowest setting. If you would like to buy a new deodorant tube please see resource section. Use an oven mitt to protect your hand, hold the deodorant tube over the garbage can then pour liquid into the tube. Place cap on the top of tube and keep in the refrigerator overnight until liquid solidifies.

To Use:

Apply to underarms.

Note: This recipe is a deodorant not a antiperspirant.

{Deodorant}

Ingredients:

1/2 cup coconut oil
1/4 cup cornstarch
1/4 cup baking soda
15 drops tea tree essential oil

Directions:

Scoop coconut oil into a microwave safe bowl with pour spout. Microwave in 30 second increments at 50 percent power, stirring each time, until it mostly liquid. Remove bowl with an oven mitt. Stir in coconut oil until clear, not cloudy. Let cool slightly, then stir in additional ingredients.

Create a tight seal at the bottom of an empty deodorant tube by screwing canister to its lowest setting. If you would like to buy a new deodorant tube please see resource section. Use an oven mitt to protect your hand, hold the deodorant tube over the garbage can then pour liquid into the tube. Place cap on the top of tube and keep in the refrigerator overnight until liquid solidifies.

To Use:

Apply to underarms.

Note: This recipe is a deodorant not a antiperspirant.

Healing Salves

{Sunburn Healing Salve}

Ingredients:

1/2 cup of raw organic honey
6 drops of Lavender essential oil
2 tsp of organic Beeswax (shredded)
2 tsp organic Aloe Vera gel

Tools Needed:

Double Boiler

A Wooden Spoon

Grater for Beeswax

4-ounce Glass Jar

Directions:

Step 1: Use a very low heat and but the beeswax into a double boiler. When melted, put the remaining ingredients in the double boiler and mix until they are thoroughly combined and there are no lumps or clumps.

Step 2: Take the pan off the double boiler and pour into

chosen container(s). It will take about a half hour to cool before you can start using it. About 7 to 9 hours.

How to Use:

Apply to sunburned areas.

{Honey Healing Salve For Cuts}

Ingredients:

1 tbsp of raw organic honey
2 drops of Green Tea Essential oil
1 drop of Tea Tree Oil
1/2 tsp of shaven beeswax

Tools Needed:

Double Boiler

A Wooden Spoon

Grater for Beeswax

4-ounce Glass Jar

Directions:

Step 1: Use a very low heat and but the beeswax into a double boiler. When melted, put the remaining ingredients in the double boiler and mix until they are thoroughly combined and there are no lumps or clumps.

Step 2: Take the pan off the double boiler and pour into chosen container(s). It will take about a half hour to cool before you can start using it. About 3 hours.

How to Use:

Apply to small cuts. Seek medical attention if you have a deep cut that may require stitches or if you have excessive bleeding that will not stop.

{Dry Skin Moisturizing Salve}

Ingredients:

2 tbsp of beeswax
4 drops of Chamomile Essential Oil
1 Vitamin E capsule squeezed
4 drops of Lavender Essential Oil

Tools Needed:

Double Boiler

A Wooden Spoon

Grater for Beeswax

6-ounce Glass Jar

Directions:

Step 1: Use a very low heat and but the beeswax into a double boiler. When melted, put the remaining ingredients in the double boiler and mix until they are thoroughly combined and there are no lumps or clumps.

Step 2: Take the pan off the double boiler and pour into

chosen container(s). It will take about a half hour to cool before you can start using it. About 4 hours.

How to Use:

Apply to areas that need moisturizing such as knees, elbows, hands, arms, legs.

Solid Perfume

{Customizable Solid Perfume}

Ingredients:

2 tbsp grated beeswax or beeswax pastilles
2 tsp jojoba oil
10 drops roman chamomile essential oil
4 drops orange essential oil
10 drops lavender essential oil

Directions:

Mix beeswax into a microwave safe bowl with a pour spout. Microwave in 30 second increments at 50 percent power, stirring each time, until it becomes liquid. Remove bowl with an oven mitt and stir until clear. Add jojoba oil and essential oils and stir. Immediately pour into container of your choice. Let harden at room temperature. This recipe makes about 1 tablespoon. Store in a cool, dry place.

To Use:

Apply a small amount to inner wrists and behind the ears.

Note: Have fun and create your own unique scent by mixing essential oils.

Sunscreen

{Aloe Vera and Coconut Oil}

Aloe vera is a good active ingredient to reach for in your homemade sunscreen arsenal. It's been proved to both treat and prevent burns on your skin.

Note: This recipe isn't waterproof, and it'll need to be reapplied often.

Ingredients
- 1/4 cup coconut oil (has an SPF of 7)
- 2 (or more) tbsp. powdered zinc oxide
- 1/4 cup pure aloe vera gel
- 1 cup (or less) shea butter

Instructions
1. Combine all ingredients, except the zinc oxide and aloe vera gel, in a medium saucepan. Let the shea butter and oils melt together at medium heat.
2. Let cool for several minutes before stirring in aloe vera gel.
3. Cool completely before adding zinc oxide. Mix well to make sure the zinc oxide is distributed throughout. You may want to add some beeswax or another waxy substance for a stickier consistency.

Store in a glass jar, and keep in a cool, dry place until you're ready to use.

Tooth Paste & Mouth Wash

{Minty Tooth Paste}

Ingredients:

1/3 cup coconut oil
1/3 cup baking soda
1/4 tsp stevia extract powder

Directions:

Melt coconut oil in microwaveable safe bowl in 10 second increments at 50 percent power, stirring in between. Remove from microwave with oven mitt. Stir in baking soda and stevia.

To turn the liquid into a paste, cover the bowl with plastic wrap and place in the refrigerator until the liquid resembles softened butter. Add essential oil, then whip with a hand mixer on low speed for 3-5 minutes, or until the color brightens and peaks form. Store in a lidded container in a cool dry place.

To Use:

Place tooth paste on your toothbrush. Brush for two minutes. Rinse mouth when completed. Do not swallow.

Note: The toothpaste will dissolve while brushing your teeth.

{Peppermint Mouthwash}

Ingredients:

4 tbsp distilled water
1/4 tsp baking soda
1/8 tsp salt
1/8 tsp stevia extract powder for sweetness (optional)
1-2 drops peppermint essential oil

Directions:

Mix all ingredients in a bowel with a pour spout. Pour into a lidded bottle. Makes enough to fill a 2 ounce bottle. Store in a cool, dry place.

To Use:

Swish around in your mouth for 30 seconds then spit into sink. Do not swallow.

Chapter 5: Bonus Recipes

Laundry Detergent

{Homemade Laundry Detergent}

Ingredients:

1 bar (or 4.5 ounces) shaved bar soap (a handmade laundry bar, Dr. Bronner's, Kirk's Castile Soap, Ivory, ZOTE, or Fels-Naptha)

1 cup borax
1 cup washing soda

Directions:

Step 1: Thoroughly stir together for several minutes.

Step 2: Store in a sealed container with a small scoop.

Notes:

Each batch yields approximately 32 ounces (between 32-64 loads based on how many Tbsp used per load).

Use 1 Tbsp per small load (or 2-3 Tbsp for large or heavily soiled loads).

Scented Sprays

{Pillow Spray}

Ingredients:

3 tbsp distilled water
1 tsp witch hazel
5 drops lavender essential oil
10 drops roman chamomile essential oil

Directions:

Mix all ingredients in a bowl with a pour spout. Pour into a spray bottle. Each recipe makes enough to fill a 2 ounce container.

To Use:

Spritz on pillows

{Citrus Linen Spray}

Ingredients:

3 tbsp distilled water
1 tsp witch hazel
15 drops lemon essential oil

Directions:

Mix all ingredients in a bowl with a pour spout. Pour into a spray bottle. Each recipe makes enough to fill a 2 ounce container.

To Use:

Spritz on linens

Chapter 6: Resources

Sourcing Materials

Amazon - www.amazon.com

Brambleberry.com - www.brambleberry.com

Bulk Apothecary.com - www.bulkapothecary.com

FDA-www.fda.gov/cosmetics/labeling/default.htm

From Nature with Love - www.fromnaturewithlove.com

Making Cosmetics - www.makingcosmetics.com

Rose Mountain Herbs - www.mountainroseherbs.com

The Chemistry Store - www.thechemistrystore.com

The Herbarie - www.theherbarie.com

Wholesale Supplies Plus - www.wholesalesuppliesplus.com

Packaging Materials

Brambleberry.com - www.brambleberry.com

Bulk Apothecary.com - www.bulkapothecary.com

FDA-www.fda.gov/cosmetics/labeling/default.htm

Rose Mountain Herbs - www.mountainroseherbs.com

Making Cosmetics - www.makingcosmetics.com

Wholesale Supplies Plus - www.wholesalesuppliesplus.com

Conclusion

Thank you for taking the time to read my book! If you follow the suggestions and recipes I have shown you in this book, you will be well on your way to starting your own home apothecary.

Take extra time to educate yourself and take courses offered by the resources listed in this book. Learn about the products, ingredients, and industry if you choose to pursue this as a small home-based business. Make a commitment to yourself to use quality products and ingredients.

Now go and whip up some fabulous handmade products!

About The Author

Kimberly Hodge

As an entrepreneur, Kimberly has shown that she has what it takes to start a home-based business and make it a success.

After starting several successful businesses, including an all-natural bath and body and candle company for many years, she now shares her creative knowledge with her readers.

Kimberly is a Licensed Massage Therapist (LMT), retired health and wellness instructor, and a yoga practitioner.

She has a vast amount of knowledge in entrepreneurial business, small business start-ups, owning and operating a successful business. Her writing focuses on health and wellness topics, business, and spiritual subjects. When she is not writing, she enjoys spending time with her husband and their fur baby and practicing yoga.

Books By This Author

Bath & Body Business: A Girl's Guide To Starting A Homebased Business

This book was written by an experienced business owner who shares her creative path to starting a successful business from home. You will learn the basics to get you up and running quickly and efficiently.

Anxiety: Find Relief Naturally

Find Peace from Anxiety Naturally and Transform Your Life.

Simply Handmade: Handcrafted Beauty & Skincare Recipes

You will learn the basics needed to start your own home apothecary using safe and accessible ingredients creating your own handcrafted bath and body products.

Appendix

Chapter 1: Basic Skincare

Bath & Body Business: A Girl's Guide to Starting a Home-based Business, Kimberly Hodge

The Ultimate Beginner's Guide to Skincare, Allure.com
https://www.allure.com/story/beginner-skin-care-routine

Small Business & Homemade Cosmetics Fact Sheet, FDA
https://www.fda.gov/cosmetics/resources-industry-cosmetics/small-businesses-homemade-cosmetics-fact-sheet

Chapter 2: Getting Started

Bath & Body Business: A Girl's Guide to Starting a Home-based Business, Kimberly Hodge

All About Citric Acid in Cosmetic & Personal Care, New Directions Aromatic,
https://www.newdirectionsaromatics.com/blog/products/all-about-citric-acid-in-cosmetics-personal-care.html

Small Business & Homemade Cosmetics Fact Sheet, FDA
https://www.fda.gov/cosmetics/resources-industry-cosmetics/small-businesses-homemade-cosmetics-fact-sheet

Flammable Liquid, Electronic Code of Federal Regulations, Cornell Law School, https://www.law.cornell.edu/cfr/text/49/173.120

Cosmetics & U.S. Law,
https://www.fda.gov/cosmetics/cosmetics-laws-regulations/
cosmetics-us-law

Cosmetic Info, Cosmeticinfo.org
https://www.cosmeticsinfo.org/

Chapter 3: Home Apothecary

Bath & Body Business: A Girl's Guide to Starting a Home-based Business, Kimberly Hodge

Chapter 4: Skincare Recipes

Bath & Body Business: A Girl's Guide to Starting a Home-based Business, Kimberly Hodge

Healing Salves, Karina Wilde
Www.thefruitfulmind.com
Botanical Beauty, Switch Press, Aubre Andrus

The Natural Beauty Recipe Book, Stephanie Rose

The Coconut Oil Cure, Essential Recipes and Remedies to Heal Your Body Inside and Out, Fall River Press

Chapter 5: Bonus Recipes

Bath & Body Business: A Girl's Guide to Starting a Home-based Business, Kimberly Hodge

Chapter 6: Resources

Brambleberry.com - www.brambleberry.com

Bulk Apothecary.com - www.bulkapothecary.com

Rose Mountain Herbs - www.mountainroseherbs.com

Connect With The Author

To connect with Kimberly and receive the latest updates on newly published books:

Website: www.kimberlyhodgebooks.com
Facebook: www.facebook.com/kimberlyhodgebooks
Twitter: www.twitter.com/kimhodgebooks
Pinterest: www.pinterest.com/kimberlyhodgebooks/
Instagram: www.instagram.com/kimberlyhodgebooks

*If you see any spelling errors in this book please email us so that we can make a correction.